GLOBAL INITIATIVE FOR CHRONIC OBSTRUCTIVE LUNG DISEASE

POCKET GUIDE TO COPD DIAGNOSIS, MANAGEMENT, AND PREVENTION
A Guide for Health Care Professionals
2017 EDITION

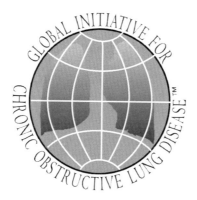

TABLE OF CONTENTS

TABLE OF CONTENTS IV

GLOBAL STRATEGY FOR THE DIAGNOSIS,
MANAGEMENT, AND PREVENTION OF COPD...... 1

INTRODUCTION 1

DEFINITION AND OVERVIEW............................ 1

OVERALL KEY POINTS: 1
WHAT IS CHRONIC OBSTRUCTIVE PULMONARY 2
DISEASE (COPD)?.. 2
WHAT CAUSES COPD?...................................... 2

DIAGNOSIS AND ASSESSMENT OF COPD............. 4

OVERALL KEY POINTS: 4
DIAGNOSIS 4
DIFFERENTIAL DIAGNOSIS 5
ASSESSMENT.. 6
*Classification of severity of airflow
obstruction* 6
Assessment of symptoms 6
Revised combined COPD assessment 8

EVIDENCE SUPPORTING PREVENTION AND
MAINTENANCE THERAPY 10

OVERALL KEY POINTS: 10
SMOKING CESSATION 11
VACCINATIONS.. 11
Influenza vaccine... 11
Pneumococcal vaccine 11
PHARMACOLOGIC THERAPY FOR STABLE COPD
.... 12
Bronchodilators.. 12
Beta$_2$-agonists.. 12
Antimuscarinic drugs.................................... 13
Methylxanthines.. 13
Combination bronchodilator therapy......... 13
Anti-inflammatory agents 16
Inhaled corticosteroids (ICS)...................... 16
Issues related to inhaled delivery 18
Other pharmacologic treatments................. 19
REHABILITATION, EDUCATION & SELF-
MANAGEMENT 20
Pulmonary rehabilitation 20
SUPPORTIVE, PALLIATIVE, END-OF-LIFE &
HOSPICE CARE.. 20
Symptom control and palliative care 20
OTHER TREATMENTS 21

Oxygen therapy and ventilatory support.... 21

MANAGEMENT OF STABLE COPD 24

OVERALL KEY POINTS: 24
IDENTIFY AND REDUCE EXPOSURE TO RISK
FACTORS.. 24
TREATMENT OF STABLE COPD......................... 25
PHARMACOLOGIC TREATMENT................... 25
Pharmacologic treatment algorithms 27
MONITORING AND FOLLOW-UP....................... 30

MANAGEMENT OF EXACERBATIONS 31

OVERALL KEY POINTS: 31
TREATMENT OPTIONS 32
HOSPITAL DISCHARGE AND FOLLOW-UP......... 36

COPD AND COMORBIDITIES 38

OVERALL KEY POINTS:................................. 38
REFERENCES 39

GLOBAL STRATEGY FOR THE DIAGNOSIS, MANAGEMENT, AND PREVENTION OF COPD

INTRODUCTION

Chronic Obstructive Pulmonary Disease (COPD) represents an important public health challenge and is a major cause of chronic morbidity and mortality throughout the world. COPD is currently the fourth leading cause of death in the world[1] but is projected to be the 3rd leading cause of death by 2020. More than 3 million people died of COPD in 2012 accounting for 6% of all deaths globally. Globally, the COPD burden is projected to increase in coming decades because of continued exposure to COPD risk factors and aging of the population.[2]

This Pocket Guide has been developed from the *Global Strategy for the Diagnosis, Management, and Prevention of COPD* (2017 Report), which aims to provide a non-biased review of the current evidence for the assessment, diagnosis and treatment of patients with COPD that can aid the clinician. Discussions of COPD and COPD management, evidence levels, and specific citations from the scientific literature are included in that source document, which is available from www.goldcopd.org. The tables and figures in this Pocket Guide follow the numbering of the 2017 Global Strategy Report for reference consistency.

DEFINITION AND OVERVIEW

OVERALL KEY POINTS:

- *Chronic Obstructive Pulmonary Disease (COPD) is a common, preventable and treatable disease that is characterized by persistent respiratory symptoms and airflow limitation that is due to airway and/or alveolar abnormalities usually caused by significant exposure to noxious particles or gases.*

- *The most common respiratory symptoms include dyspnea, cough and/or sputum production. These symptoms may be under-reported by patients.*

- *The main risk factor for COPD is tobacco smoking but other environmental exposures such as biomass fuel exposure and air pollution may contribute. Besides exposures, host factors predispose individuals to develop COPD. These include genetic abnormalities, abnormal lung development and accelerated aging.*

- *COPD may be punctuated by periods of acute worsening of respiratory symptoms, called exacerbations.*

- *In most patients, COPD is associated with significant concomitant chronic diseases, which increase its morbidity and mortality.*

WHAT IS CHRONIC OBSTRUCTIVE PULMONARY DISEASE (COPD)?

Chronic Obstructive Pulmonary Disease (COPD) is a common, preventable and treatable disease that is characterized by persistent respiratory symptoms and airflow limitation that is due to airway and/or alveolar abnormalities usually caused by significant exposure to noxious particles or gases. The chronic airflow limitation that is characteristic of COPD is caused by a mixture of small airways disease (e.g., obstructive bronchiolitis) and parenchymal destruction (emphysema), the relative contributions of which vary from person to person (**Figure 1.1**).

Figure 1.1. Etiology, pathobiology and pathology of COPD leading to airflow limitation and clinical manifestations

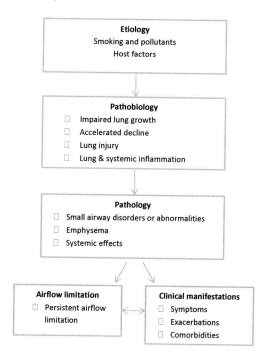

WHAT CAUSES COPD?

Worldwide, the most commonly encountered risk factor for COPD is **tobacco smoking**. Other types of tobacco, (e.g. pipe, cigar, water pipe) and marijuana are also risk factors for COPD. Outdoor, occupational, and indoor air pollution – the latter resulting from the burning of biomass fuels – are other major COPD risk factors.

Nonsmokers may also develop COPD. COPD is the result of a complex interplay of long-term cumulative exposure to noxious gases and particles, combined with a variety of host factors including genetics, airway hyper-responsiveness and poor lung growth during childhood.[3-5]

Often, the prevalence of COPD is directly related to the prevalence of tobacco smoking, although in many countries outdoor, occupational and indoor air pollution (resulting from the burning of wood and other biomass fuels) are major COPD risk factors.[6,7]

The risk of developing COPD is related to the following factors:

- **Tobacco smoke** - including cigarette, pipe, cigar, water-pipe and other types of tobacco smoking popular in many countries, as well as environmental tobacco smoke (ETS)

- **Indoor air pollution** - from biomass fuel used for cooking and heating in poorly vented dwellings, a risk factor that particularly affects women in developing countries

- **Occupational exposures** - including organic and inorganic dusts, chemical agents and fumes, are under-appreciated risk factors for COPD.[6,8]

- **Outdoor air pollution** - also contributes to the lungs' total burden of inhaled particles, although it appears to have a relatively small effect in causing COPD.

- **Genetic factors** - such as severe hereditary deficiency of alpha-1 antitrypsin (AATD).[9]

- **Age and gender** - aging and female gender increase COPD risk.

- **Lung growth and development** - any factor that affects lung growth during gestation and childhood (low birth weight, respiratory infections, etc.) has the potential to increase an individual's risk of developing COPD.

- **Socioeconomic status** - there is strong evidence that the risk of developing COPD is inversely related to socioeconomic status.[10] It is not clear, however, whether this pattern reflects exposures to indoor and outdoor air pollutants, crowding, poor nutrition, infections, or other factors related to low socioeconomic status.

- **Asthma and airway hyper-reactivity** - asthma may be a risk factor for the development of airflow limitation and COPD.

- **Chronic bronchitis** - may increase the frequency of total and severe exacerbations.

- **Infections** - a history of severe childhood respiratory infection has been associated with reduced lung function and increased respiratory symptoms in adulthood.[11]

DIAGNOSIS AND ASSESSMENT OF COPD

OVERALL KEY POINTS:

• *COPD should be considered in any patient who has dyspnea, chronic cough or sputum production, and/or a history of exposure to risk factors for the disease.*

• *Spirometry is required to make the diagnosis; the presence of a post-bronchodilator $FEV_1/FVC < 0.70$ confirms the presence of persistent airflow limitation.*

• *The goals of COPD assessment are to determine the severity of the disease, including the severity of airflow limitation, the impact of disease on the patient's health status, and the risk of future events (such as exacerbations, hospital admissions, or death), in order to guide therapy.*

• *Concomitant chronic diseases occur frequently in COPD patients, including cardiovascular disease, skeletal muscle dysfunction, metabolic syndrome, osteoporosis, depression, anxiety, and lung cancer. These comorbidities should be actively sought and treated appropriately when present as they can influence mortality and hospitalizations independently.*

DIAGNOSIS

COPD should be considered in any patient who has dyspnea, chronic cough or sputum production, and/or history of exposure to risk factors for the disease. A detailed medical history of a new patient who is known, or suspected, to have COPD is essential. Spirometry is required to make the diagnosis in this clinical context[12]; the presence of a post-bronchodilator $FEV_1/FVC < 0.70$ confirms the presence of persistent airflow limitation and thus of COPD in patients with appropriate symptoms and significant exposures to noxious stimuli. Spirometry is the most reproducible and objective measurement of airflow limitation. It is a noninvasive and readily available test. Despite its good sensitivity, peak expiratory flow measurement alone cannot be reliably used as the only diagnostic test because of its weak specificity.[13]

Table 2.1. Key indicators for considering a diagnosis of COPD	
Consider COPD, and perform spirometry, if any of these indicators are present in an individual over age 40. These indicators are not diagnostic themselves, but the presence of multiple key indicators increases the probability of a diagnosis of COPD. Spirometry is required to establish a diagnosis of COPD.	
Dyspnea that is:	Progressive over time.
	Characteristically worse with exercise.
	Persistent.
Chronic cough:	May be intermittent and may be unproductive.
	Recurrent wheeze.
Chronic sputum production:	Any pattern of chronic sputum production may indicate COPD.
Recurrent lower respiratory tract infections	
History of risk factors:	Host factors (such as genetic factors,

	congenital/developmental abnormalities etc.). Tobacco smoke (including popular local preparations). Smoke from home cooking and heating fuels. Occupational dusts, vapors, fumes, gases and other chemicals.
Family history of COPD and/or childhood factors:	For example low birthweight, childhood respiratory infections etc.

DIFFERENTIAL DIAGNOSIS

A major differential diagnosis is asthma. In some patients with chronic asthma, a clear distinction from COPD is not possible using current imaging and physiological testing techniques. In these patients, current management is similar to that of asthma. Other potential diagnoses are usually easier to distinguish from COPD (**Table 2.7**).

Table 2.7. Differential diagnosis of COPD	
Diagnosis	**Suggestive Features**
COPD	Onset in mid-life. Symptoms slowly progressive. History of tobacco smoking or exposure to other types of smoke.
Asthma	Onset early in life (often childhood). Symptoms vary widely from day to day. Symptoms worse at night/early morning. Allergy, rhinitis, and/or eczema also present. Family history of asthma. Obesity coexistence.
Congestive Heart Failure	Chest X-ray shows dilated heart, pulmonary edema. Pulmonary function tests indicate volume restriction, not airflow
Bronchiectasis	Large volumes of purulent sputum. Commonly associated with bacterial infection. Chest X-ray/CT shows bronchial dilation, bronchial wall thickening.
Tuberculosis	Onset all ages. Chest X-ray shows lung infiltrate. Microbiological confirmation. High local prevalence of tuberculosis.
Obliterative Bronchiolitis	Onset at younger age, nonsmokers. May have history of rheumatoid arthritis or acute fume exposure. Seen after lung or bone marrow transplantation. CT on expiration shows hypodense areas.
Diffuse Panbronchiolitis	Predominantly seen in patients of Asian descent. Most patients are male and nonsmokers. Almost all have chronic sinusitis. Chest X-ray and HRCT show diffuse small centrilobular nodular opacities and hyperinflation.
These features tend to be characteristic of the respective diseases, but are not mandatory. For example, a person who has never smoked may develop COPD (especially in the developing world where other risk factors may be more important than cigarette smoking); asthma may develop in adult and even in elderly patients.	

Alpha-1 antitrypsin deficiency (AATD) screening. The World Health Organization recommends that all patients with a diagnosis of COPD should be screened once especially in areas with high AATD prevalence.[14] A low concentration (< 20% normal) is highly suggestive of homozygous deficiency. Family members should also be screened.

ASSESSMENT

The goals of COPD assessment are to determine the severity of airflow limitation, its impact on the patient's health status and the risk of future events (such as exacerbations, hospital admissions or death), in order to, eventually, guide therapy. To achieve these goals, COPD assessment must consider the following aspects of the disease separately:

- The presence and severity of the spirometric abnormality
- Current nature and magnitude of the patient's symptoms
- Exacerbation history and future risk
- Presence of comorbidities

Classification of severity of airflow obstruction

The classification of airflow limitation severity in COPD is shown in **Table 2.4**. Specific spirometric cut-points are used for purposes of simplicity. Spirometry should be performed after the administration of an adequate dose of at least one short-acting inhaled bronchodilator in order to minimize variability.

Table 2.4. Classification of airflow limitation severity in COPD (based on post-bronchodilator FEV_1) In patients with $FEV_1/FVC < 0.70$:		
GOLD 1:	Mild	$FEV_1 \geq 80\%$ predicted
GOLD 2:	Moderate	$50\% \leq FEV_1 < 80\%$ predicted
GOLD 3:	Severe	$30\% \leq FEV_1 < 50\%$ predicted
GOLD 4:	Very Severe	$FEV_1 < 30\%$ predicted

It should be noted that there is only a weak correlation between FEV_1, symptoms and impairment of a patient's health status.[15,16] For this reason, formal symptomatic assessment is also required.

Assessment of symptoms

In the past, COPD was viewed as a disease largely characterized by breathlessness. A simple measure of breathlessness such as the Modified British Medical Research Council (mMRC) Questionnaire[17] **(Table 2.5)** was considered adequate, as the mMRC relates well to other measures of health status and predicts future mortality risk.[18,19]

Table 2.5. Modified MRC dyspnea scale[a]	
PLEASE TICK IN THE BOX THAT APPLIES TO YOU (ONE BOX ONLY) (Grades 0-4)	
mMRC Grade 0. I only get breathless with strenuous exercise.	❑
mMRC Grade 1. I get short of breath when hurrying on the level or walking up a slight hill.	❑
mMRC Grade 2. I walk slower than people of the same age on the level because of breathlessness, or I have to stop for breath when walking on my own pace on the level.	❑
mMRC Grade 3. I stop for breath after walking about 100 meters or after a few minutes on the level.	❑
mMRC Grade 4. I am too breathless to leave the house or I am breathless when dressing or undressing.	❑

[a] Fletcher CM. BMJ 1960; 2: 1662.

Figure 2.3. CAT Assessment

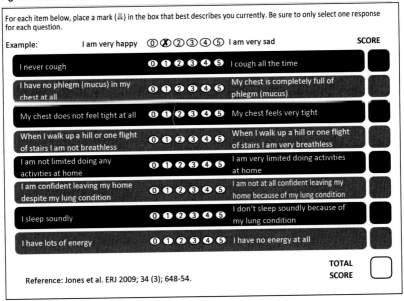

Reference: Jones et al. ERJ 2009; 34 (3); 648-54.

However, it is now recognized that COPD impacts patients beyond just dyspnea.[20] For this reason, a comprehensive assessment of symptoms is recommended using measures such as the COPD Assessment Test (CAT™)[1] (**Figure 2.3**) and the COPD Control Questionnaire (The CCQ©) have been developed and are suitable.

[1] The COPD Assessment Test was developed by a multi-disciplinary group of international experts in COPD supported by GSK. COPD Assessment Test and the CAT logo is a trademark of the GlaxoSmithKline group of companies. © 2009 GlaxoSmithKline. All rights reserved. GSK activities with respect to the COPD Assessment Test are overseen by a governance board that includes independent external experts, one of whom chairs the board.

Revised combined COPD assessment

An understanding of the impact of COPD on an individual patient combines the symptomatic assessment with the patient's spirometric classification and/or risk of exacerbations. The "ABCD" assessment tool of the 2011 GOLD update was a major advancement from the simple spirometric grading system of the earlier versions of GOLD because it incorporated patient-reported outcomes and highlighted the importance of exacerbation prevention in the management of COPD. However, there were some important limitations. Firstly, the ABCD assessment tool performed no better than the spirometric grades for mortality prediction or other important health outcomes in COPD.[21-23] Moreover, group "D" outcomes were modified by two parameters: lung function and/or exacerbation history, which caused confusion.[16] To address these and other concerns (while at the same time maintaining consistency and simplicity for the practicing clinician), a refinement of the ABCD assessment tool is proposed that separates spirometric grades from the "ABCD" groups. For some therapeutic recommendations, ABCD groups will be derived exclusively from patient symptoms and their history of exacerbation. Spirometry in conjunction with patient symptoms and exacerbation history remains vital for the diagnosis, prognostication and consideration of other important therapeutic approaches. This new approach to assessment is illustrated in **Figure 2.4.**

In the refined assessment scheme, patients should undergo spirometry to determine the severity of airflow limitation (i.e., spirometric grade). They should then undergo assessment of either dyspnea using mMRC or symptoms using CAT™. Finally, their history of exacerbations (including prior hospitalizations) should be recorded.

Figure 2.4. The refined ABCD assessment tool

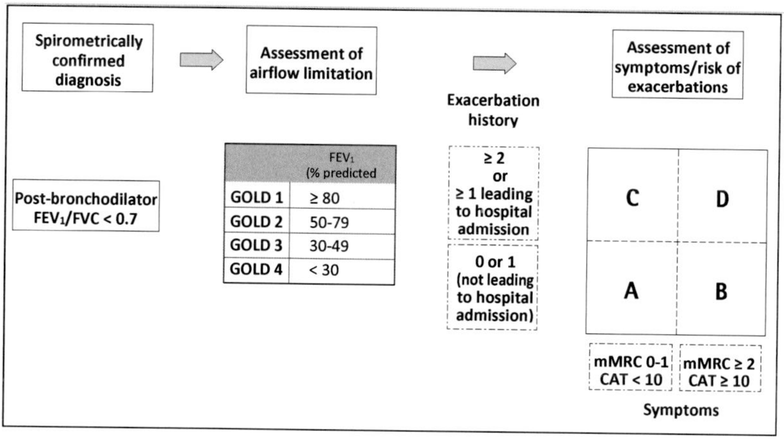

Example: Consider two patients - both patients with $FEV_1 < 30\%$ of predicted, CAT scores of 18 and one with no exacerbations in the past year and the other with three exacerbations in the past year. Both would have been labelled GOLD D in the prior classification scheme. However, with the new proposed scheme, the subject with 3 exacerbations in the past year would be labelled GOLD grade 4, group D; the other subject with no exacerbations would be labelled GOLD Grade 4, group B.

This classification scheme may facilitate consideration of individual therapies (exacerbation prevention versus symptom relief as outlined in the above example) and also help guide escalation and de-escalation therapeutic strategies for a specific patient.

EVIDENCE SUPPORTING PREVENTION AND MAINTENANCE THERAPY

OVERALL KEY POINTS:

- *Smoking cessation is key. Pharmacotherapy and nicotine replacement reliably increase long-term smoking abstinence rates.*

- *The effectiveness and safety of e-cigarettes as a smoking cessation aid is uncertain at present.*

- *Pharmacologic therapy can reduce COPD symptoms, reduce the frequency and severity of exacerbations, and improve health status and exercise tolerance.*

- *Each pharmacologic treatment regimen should be individualized and guided by the severity of symptoms, risk of exacerbations, side-effects, comorbidities, drug availability and cost, and the patient's response, preference and ability to use various drug delivery devices.*

- *Inhaler technique needs to be assessed regularly.*

- *Influenza vaccination decreases the incidence of lower respiratory tract infections.*

- *Pneumococcal vaccination decreases lower respiratory tract infections.*

- *Pulmonary rehabilitation improves symptoms, quality of life, and physical and emotional participation in everyday activities.*

- *In patients with severe resting chronic hypoxemia, long-term oxygen therapy improves survival.*

- *In patients with stable COPD and resting or exercise-induced moderate desaturation, long-term oxygen treatment should not be prescribed routinely. However, individual patient factors must be considered when evaluating the patient's need for supplemental oxygen.*

- *In patients with severe chronic hypercapnia and a history of hospitalization for acute respiratory failure, long-term non-invasive ventilation may decrease mortality and prevent re-hospitalization.*

- *In select patients with advanced emphysema refractory to optimized medical care, surgical or bronchoscopic interventional treatments may be beneficial.*

- *Palliative approaches are effective in controlling symptoms in advanced COPD.*

SMOKING CESSATION

Smoking cessation has the greatest capacity to influence the natural history of COPD. If effective resources and time are dedicated to smoking cessation, long-term quit success rates of up to 25% can be achieved.[24]

A five-step program for intervention (**Table 3.1**)[25-27] provides a helpful strategic framework to guide health care providers interested in helping their patients stop smoking.[25,27,28]

Table 3.1. Brief strategies to help the patient willing to quit	
• **ASK:**	Systematically identify all tobacco users at every visit.
	Implement an office-wide system that ensures that, for EVERY patient at EVERY clinic visit, tobacco-use status is queried and documented.
• **ADVISE:**	Strongly urge all tobacco users to quit.
	In a clear, strong, and personalized manner, urge every tobacco user to quit.
• **ASSESS:**	Determine willingness and rationale of patient's desire to make a quit attempt.
	Ask every tobacco user if he or she is willing to make a quit attempt at this time (e.g., within the next 30 days).
• **ASSIST:**	Aid the patient in quitting.
	Help the patient with a quit plan; provide practical counseling; provide intra-treatment social support; help the patient obtain extra-treatment social support; recommend use of approved pharmacotherapy except in special circumstances; provide supplementary materials.
• **ARRANGE:**	Schedule follow-up contact.
	Schedule follow-up contact, either in person or via telephone.

Counseling. Counseling delivered by physicians and other health professionals significantly increases quit rates over self-initiated strategies.[29] Even brief (3-minute) periods of counseling urging a smoker to quit improve smoking cessation rates.[29] There is a relationship between counseling intensity and cessation success.[30]

VACCINATIONS

Influenza vaccine

Influenza vaccination can reduce serious illness (such as lower respiratory tract infections requiring hospitalization)[31] and death in COPD patients.[32-35]

Pneumococcal vaccine

Pneumococcal vaccinations, PCV13 and PPSV23, are recommended for all patients ≥ 65 years of age (**Table 3.2**). The PPSV23 is also recommended for younger COPD patients with significant comorbid conditions including chronic heart or lung disease.[36] PPSV23 has been shown to reduce the incidence of community-acquired pneumonia in COPD patients < 65 years, with an FEV_1 < 40% predicted, or comorbidities (especially cardiac comorbidities).[37]

Table 3.2. Vaccination for stable COPD

- Influenza vaccination reduces serious illness and death in COPD patients (**Evidence B**).
- The 23-valent pneumococcal polysaccharide vaccine (PPSV23) has been shown to reduce the incidence of community- acquired pneumonia in COPD patients aged < 65 years with an FEV1 < 40% predicted and in those with comorbidities (**Evidence B**).
- In the general population of adults ≥ 65 years the 13-valent conjugated pneumococcal vaccine (PCV13) has demonstrated significant efficacy in reducing bacteremia and serious invasive pneumococcal disease (**Evidence B**).

PHARMACOLOGIC THERAPY FOR STABLE COPD

Pharmacologic therapy for COPD is used to reduce symptoms, reduce the frequency and severity of exacerbations, and improve exercise tolerance and health status. To date, there is no conclusive clinical trial evidence that any existing medications for COPD modify the long-term decline in lung function.[38-42]

The classes of medications commonly used to treat COPD are shown in **Table 3.3**.

Bronchodilators

Bronchodilators are medications that increase FEV_1 and/or change other spirometric variables.

- Bronchodilator medications in COPD are most often given on a regular basis to prevent or reduce symptoms.
- Toxicity is also dose-related (**Table 3.3**).
- Use of short acting bronchodilators on a regular basis is not generally recommended.

Beta$_2$-agonists

- The principal action of beta$_2$-agonists is to relax airway smooth muscle by stimulating beta$_2$-adrenergic receptors, which increases cyclic AMP and produces functional antagonism to bronchoconstriction.
- There are short-acting (SABA) and long-acting (LABA) beta$_2$-agonists.
- Formoterol and salmeterol are twice-daily LABAs that significantly improve FEV_1 and lung volumes, dyspnea, health status, exacerbation rate and number of hospitalizations, [43] but have no effect on mortality or rate of decline of lung function.
- Indacaterol is a once daily LABA that improves breathlessness,[44,45] health status[45] and exacerbation rate.[45]
- Oladaterol and vilanterol are additional once daily LABAs that improve lung function and

12

symptoms.[46,47]

- *Adverse effects.* Stimulation of beta$_2$-adrenergic receptors can produce resting sinus tachycardia and has the potential to precipitate cardiac rhythm disturbances in susceptible patients. Exaggerated somatic tremor is troublesome in some older patients treated with higher doses of beta$_2$-agonists, regardless of route of administration.

Antimuscarinic drugs

- Antimuscarinic drugs block the bronchoconstrictor effects of acetylcholine on M3 muscarinic receptors expressed in airway smooth muscle.[48]
- Short-acting antimuscarinics (SAMAs), namely ipratropium and oxitropium and long-acting antimuscarinic antagonists (LAMAs), such as tiotropium, aclidinium, glycopyrronium bromide and umeclidinium act on the receptors in different ways.[48]
- A systematic review of RCTs found that ipratropium alone provided small benefits over short-acting beta$_2$-agonist in terms of lung function, health status and requirement for oral steroids.[49]
- Clinical trials have shown a greater effect on exacerbation rates for LAMA treatment (tiotropium) versus LABA treatment.[50,51]
- *Adverse effects.* Inhaled anticholinergic drugs are poorly absorbed which limits the troublesome systemic effects observed with atropine.[48,52] Extensive use of this class of agents in a wide range of doses and clinical settings has shown them to be very safe. The main side effect is dryness of mouth.[53,54]

Methylxanthines

- Controversy remains about the exact effects of xanthine derivatives.
- Theophylline, the most commonly used methylxanthine, is metabolized by cytochrome P450 mixed function oxidases. Clearance of the drug declines with age.
- There is evidence for a modest bronchodilator effect compared with placebo in stable COPD.[55]
- Addition of theophylline to salmeterol produces a greater improvement in FEV$_1$ and breathlessness than salmeterol alone.[56,57]
- There is limited and contradictory evidence regarding the effect of low-dose theophylline on exacerbation rates.[58,59]
- *Adverse effects.* Toxicity is dose-related, which is a particular problem with xanthine derivatives because their therapeutic ratio is small and most of the benefit occurs only when near-toxic doses are given.[55,60]

Combination bronchodilator therapy

- Combining bronchodilators with different mechanisms and durations of action may increase the degree of bronchodilation with a lower risk of side-effects compared to increasing the dose of a single bronchodilator.[61]
- Combinations of SABAs and SAMAs are superior compared to either medication alone in improving FEV$_1$ and symptoms.[62]
- Treatment with formoterol and tiotropium in *separate inhalers* has a bigger impact on FEV$_1$ than either component alone.[63]

- There are numerous combinations of a LABA and LAMA in a *single inhaler* available (**Table 3.3**).
- A lower dose, twice daily regimen for a LABA/LAMA has also been shown to improve symptoms and health status in COPD patients[64] (**Table 3.4**).

Table 3.3. Commonly used maintenance medications in COPD*

Drug	Inhaler (mcg)	Solution for nebulizer (mg/ml)	Oral	Vials for injection (mg)	Duration of action (hours)
Beta₂-agonists					
Short-acting					
Fenoterol	100-200 (MDI)	1	2.5 mg (pill), 0.05% (syrup)		4-6
Levalbuterol	45-90 (MDI)	0.1, 0.21, 0.25, 0.42			6-8
Salbutamol (albuterol)	90, 100, 200 (MDI & DPI)†	1, 2, 2.5, 5 mg/ml	2, 4, 5 mg (pill), 8 mg (extended release tablet) 0.024%/0.4 mg (syrup)	0.1, 0.5 mg	4-6, 12 (extended release)
Terbutaline	500 (DPI)		2.5, 5 mg (pill)	0.2, 0.25, 1 mg	4-6
Long-acting					
Arformoterol		0.0075†			12
Formoterol	4.5-9 (DPI)	0.01˙			12
Indacaterol	75-300 (DPI)				24
Olodaterol	2.5, 5 (SMI)				24
Salmeterol	25-50 (MDI & DPI)				12
Anticholinergics					
Short-acting					
Ipratropium bromide	20, 40 (MDI)	0.2			6-8
Oxitropium bromide	100 (MDI)				7-9
Long-acting					
Aclidinium bromide	400 (DPI), 400 (MDI)				12
Glycopyrronium bromide	15.6 & 50 (DPI)†		1 mg (solution)	0.2 mg	12-24
Tiotropium	18 (DPI), 2.5 & 5 (SMI)				24
Umeclidinium	62.5 (DPI)				24
Combination of short-acting beta₂-agonist plus anticholinergic in one device					
Fenoterol/ipratropium	50/20 (SMI)	1.25, 0.5 mg in 4ml			6-8
Salbutamol/ipratropium	100/20 (SMI), 75/15 (MDI)	0.5, 2.5 mg in 3ml			6-8
Combination of long-acting beta₂-agonist plus anticholinergic in one device					
Formoterol/aclidinium	12/400 (DPI)				12
Formoterol/glycopyrronium	9.6/14.4 (MDI)				12
Indacaterol/glycopyrronium	27.5/15.6 & 110/50 (DPI)†				12-24
Vilanterol/umeclidinium	25/62.5 (DPI)				24
Olodaterol/tiotropium	5/5 (SMI)				24
Methylxanthines					
Aminophylline			105 mg/ml (solution)	250, 500 mg	Variable, up to 24
Theophylline (SR)			100-600 mg (pill)	250, 400, 500 mg	Variable, up to 24
Combination of long-acting beta₂-agonist plus corticosteroids in one device					
Formoterol/beclomethasone	6/100 (MDI & DPI)				
Formoterol/budesonide	4.5/160 (MDI), 4.5/80 (MDI), 9/320 (DPI), 9/160 (DPI)				
Formoterol/mometasone	10/200, 10/400 (MDI)				
Salmeterol/fluticasone	5/100, 50/250, 5/500 (DPI), 21/45, 21/115, 21/230 (MDI)				
Vilanterol/fluticasone furoate	25/100 (DPI)				
Phosphodiesterase-4 inhibitors					
Roflumilast			500 mcg (pill)		

MDI – metered dose inhaler; DPI – dry powder inhaler; SMI – soft mist inhaler

* Not all formulations are available in all countries; in some countries other formulations and dosages may be available

† Dose availability varies by country

˙ Formoterol nebulized solution is based on the unit dose vial containing 20 mcg in a volume of 2.0 ml

† Dose varies by country

Table 3.4. Bronchodilators in stable COPD

- Inhaled bronchodilators in COPD are central to symptom management and commonly given on a regular basis to prevent or reduce symptoms (**Evidence A**).
- Regular and as-needed use of SABA or SAMA improves FEV1 and symptoms (**Evidence A**).
- Combinations of SABA and SAMA are superior compared to either medication alone in improving FEV1 and symptoms (**Evidence A**).
- LABAs and LAMAs significantly improve lung function, dyspnea, health status, and reduce exacerbation rates (**Evidence A**).
- LAMAs have a greater effect on exacerbation reduction compared with LABAs (**Evidence A**) and decrease hospitalizations (**Evidence B**).
- Combination treatment with a LABA and LAMA increases FEV1 and reduces symptoms compared to monotherapy (**Evidence A**).
- Combination treatment with a LABA and LAMA reduces exacerbations compared to monotherapy (**Evidence B**) or ICS/LABA (**Evidence B**).
- Tiotropium improves the effectiveness of pulmonary rehabilitation in increasing exercise performance (**Evidence B**).
- Theophylline exerts a small bronchodilator effect in stable COPD (**Evidence A**) and that is associated with modest symptomatic benefits (**Evidence B**).

Anti-inflammatory agents

- To date, exacerbations (e.g., exacerbation rate, patients with at least one exacerbation, time-to-first exacerbation) represent the main clinically relevant end-point used for efficacy assessment of drugs with anti-inflammatory effects (**Table 3.5**).

Inhaled corticosteroids (ICS)

- *ICS in combination with long-acting bronchodilator therapy.* In patients with moderate to very severe COPD and exacerbations, an ICS combined with a LABA is more effective than either component alone in improving lung function, health status and reducing exacerbations.[65,66]
- *Adverse effects.* There is high quality evidence from randomized controlled trials (RCTs) that ICS use is associated with higher prevalence of oral candidiasis, hoarse voice, skin bruising and pneumonia.[67]
- *Withdrawal of ICS.* Results from withdrawal studies provide equivocal results regarding consequences of withdrawal on lung function, symptoms and exacerbations.[68-72] Differences between studies may relate to differences in methodology, including the use of background long-acting bronchodilator medication(s) which may minimize any effect of ICS withdrawal.

Table 3.5. Anti-inflammatory therapy in stable COPD

Inhaled corticosteroids

- An ICS combined with a LABA is more effective than the individual components in improving lung function and health status and reducing exacerbations in patients with exacerbations and moderate to very severe COPD (**Evidence A**).
- Regular treatment with ICS increases the risk of pneumonia especially in those with severe disease (**Evidence A**).
- Triple inhaled therapy of ICS/LAMA/LABA improves lung function, symptoms and health status (**Evidence A**) and reduces exacerbations (**Evidence B**) compared to ICS/LABA or LAMA monotherapy.

Oral glucocorticoids

- Long-term use of oral glucocorticoids has numerous side effects (**Evidence A**) with no evidence of benefits (**Evidence C**).

PDE4 inhibitors

- In patients with chronic bronchitis, severe to very severe COPD and a history of exacerbations:
  - A PDE4 inhibitor improves lung function and reduces moderate and severe exacerbations (**Evidence A**).
  - A PDE4 inhibitor improves lung function and decreases exacerbations in patients who are on fixed-dose LABA/ICS combinations (**Evidence B**).

Antibiotics

- Long-term azithromycin and erythromycin therapy reduces exacerbations over one year (**Evidence A**).
- Treatment with azithromycin is associated with an increased incidence of bacterial resistance (**Evidence A**) and hearing test impairments (**Evidence B**).

Mucolytics/antioxidants

- Regular use of NAC and carbocysteine reduces the risk of exacerbations in select populations (**Evidence B**).

Other anti-inflammatory agents

- Simvastatin does not prevent exacerbations in COPD patients at increased risk of exacerbations and without indications for statin therapy (**Evidence A**). However, observational studies suggest that statins may have positive effects on some outcomes in patients with COPD who receive them for cardiovascular and metabolic indications (**Evidence C**).
- Leukotriene modifiers have not been tested adequately in COPD patients.

- Triple inhaled therapy
  - The step up in inhaled treatment to LABA plus LAMA plus ICS (triple therapy) can occur by various approaches.[73]
  - This may improve lung function and patient reported outcomes.[74-77]
  - Adding a LAMA to existing LABA/ICS improves lung function and patient reported outcomes, in particular exacerbation risk.[75,78-80]
  - A RCT did not demonstrate any benefit of adding ICS to LABA plus LAMA on exacerbations.[81]
  - Altogether, more evidence is needed to draw conclusions on the benefits of triple therapy LABA/LAMA/ICS compared to LABA/LAMA.

- Oral glucocorticoids
    - Oral glucocorticoids have numerous side effects, including steroid myopathy[82] which can contribute to muscle weakness, decreased functionality, and respiratory failure in subjects with very severe COPD.
    - While oral glucocorticoids play a role in the acute management of exacerbations, they have no role in the chronic daily treatment in COPD because of a lack of benefit balanced against a high rate of systemic complications.

- Phosphodiesterase-4 (PDE4) inhibitors
    - Roflumilast reduces moderate and severe exacerbations treated with systemic corticosteroids in patients with chronic bronchitis, severe to very severe COPD, and a history of exacerbations.[83]
    - *Adverse effects.* PDE4 inhibitors have more adverse effects than inhaled medications for COPD.[84] The most frequent are nausea, reduced appetite, weight loss, abdominal pain, diarrhea, sleep disturbance, and headache.

- Antibiotics
    - More recent studies have shown that regular use of macrolide antibiotics may reduce exacerbation rate.[85,86]

- Mucolytic (mucokinetics, mucoregulators) and antioxidant agents (NAC, carbocysteine)
    - In COPD patients not receiving inhaled corticosteroids, regular treatment with mucolytics such as carbocysteine and N-acetylcysteine may reduce exacerbations and modestly improve health status.[87,88]

Issues related to inhaled delivery

- Determinants of poor inhaler technique in asthma and COPD patients include: older age, use of multiple devices, and lack of previous education on inhaler technique.[89]
- The main errors in delivery device use relate to problems with inhalation rate, inhalation duration, coordination, dose preparation, exhalation maneuver prior to inhalation and breath-holding following dose inhalation (**Table 3.6**).[90]

Table 3.6. The inhaled route

- When a treatment is given by the inhaled route, the importance of education and training in inhaler device technique cannot be over-emphasized.
- The choice of inhaler device has to be individually tailored and will depend on access, cost, prescriber, and most importantly, patient's ability and preference.
- It is essential to provide instructions and to demonstrate the proper inhalation technique when prescribing a device, to ensure that inhaler technique is adequate and re-check at each visit that patients continue to use their inhaler correctly.
- Inhaler technique (and adherence to therapy) should be assessed before concluding that the current therapy is insufficient.

Other pharmacologic treatments

Other pharmacologic treatments for COPD are summarized in **Table 3.7**.

Table 3.7. Other pharmacological treatments

Alpha-1 antitrypsin augmentation therapy
- Intravenous augmentation therapy may slow down the progression of emphysema (**Evidence B**).

Antitussives
- There is no conclusive evidence of a beneficial role of antitussives in patients with COPD (**Evidence C**).

Vasodilators
- Vasodilators do not improve outcomes and may worsen oxygenation (**Evidence B**).

REHABILITATION, EDUCATION & SELF-MANAGEMENT

Pulmonary rehabilitation

- The benefits to COPD patients from pulmonary rehabilitation are considerable (**Table 3.8**), and rehabilitation has been shown to be the most effective therapeutic strategy to improve shortness of breath, health status and exercise tolerance.[91]

Table 3.8. Pulmonary rehabilitation, self-management and integrative care in COPD
Pulmonary rehabilitation
• Pulmonary rehabilitation improves dyspnea, health status and exercise tolerance in stable patients (**Evidence A**). • Pulmonary rehabilitation reduces hospitalizations among patients who have had a recent exacerbation (≤ 4 weeks from prior hospitalization) (**Evidence B**).
Education and self-management
• Education alone has not been shown to be effective (**Evidence C**). • Self-management intervention with communication with a health care professional improves health status and decreases hospitalizations and emergency department visits (**Evidence B**).
Integrated care programs
• Integrated care and telehealth have no demonstrated benefit at this time (**Evidence B**).

SUPPORTIVE, PALLIATIVE, END-OF-LIFE & HOSPICE CARE

Symptom control and palliative care

- COPD is a highly symptomatic disease and has many elements such as fatigue, dyspnea, depression, anxiety, insomnia that require symptom-based palliative treatments.
- Palliative approaches are essential in the context of end-of-life care as well as hospice care (a model for delivery of end-of-life care for patients who are terminally ill and predicted to have less than 6 months to live).

Key points for palliative, end-of-life and hospice care in COPD are summarized in **Table 3.9**.

Table 3.9. Palliative care, end of life and hospice care in COPD
Pulmonary rehabilitation
• Opiates, neuromuscular electrical stimulation (NMES), oxygen and fans blowing air onto the face can relieve breathlessness (**Evidence C**). • In malnourished patients, nutritional supplementation may improve respiratory muscle strength and overall health status (**Evidence B**). • Fatigue can be improved by self-management education, pulmonary rehabilitation, nutritional support and mind-body interventions (**Evidence B**).

OTHER TREATMENTS

Oxygen therapy and ventilatory support

Oxygen therapy.

- The long-term administration of oxygen (> 15 hours per day) to patients with chronic respiratory failure has been shown to increase survival in patients with severe resting hypoxemia (**Table 3.10**).[92]

Table 3.10. Oxygen therapy and ventilatory support in stable COPD
Oxygen therapy
• The long-term administration of oxygen increases survival in patients with severe chronic resting arterial hypoxemia (**Evidence A**).
• In patients with stable COPD and moderate resting or exercise-induced arterial desaturation, prescription of long-term oxygen does not lengthen time to death or first hospitalization or provide sustained benefit in health status, lung function and 6-minute walk distance (**Evidence A**).
• Resting oxygenation at sea level does not exclude the development of severe hypoxemia when traveling by air (**Evidence C**).
Ventilatory support
• NPPV may improve hospitalization-free survival in selected patients after recent hospitalization, particularly in those with pronounced daytime persistent hypercapnia (PaCO$_2$ ≥ 52 mmHg) (**Evidence B**).

Ventilatory support

- Noninvasive ventilation (NIV) in the form of noninvasive positive pressure ventilation (NPPV) is the standard of care for decreasing morbidity and mortality in patients hospitalized with an exacerbation of COPD and acute respiratory failure.[93-95]

Stable patient

- NPPV may improve hospitalization-free survival in selected patients after recent hospitalization, particularly in those with pronounced daytime persistent hypercapnia.[96-98]
- In patients with both COPD and obstructive sleep apnea there are clear benefits associated with the use of continuous positive airway pressure (CPAP) to improve both survival and the risk of hospital admissions.[99]

Interventional Treatments

- The advantage of lung volume reduction surgery (LVRS) over medical therapy is more significant among patients with upper-lobe predominant emphysema and low exercise capacity after rehabilitation; although LVRS is costly relative to health-care programs not including surgery.
- Non-surgical bronchoscopic lung volume reduction techniques may improve exercise tolerance, health status ans lung function in selected patients with advanced emphsyema refractory to medical therapy.

21

- In appropriately selected patients with very severe COPD, lung transplantation has been shown to improve quality of life and functional capacity.
- Key points for interventional therapy in stable COPD are summarized in **Table 3.11**, and an algorithm depicting an overview of various interventions is shown in **Figure 4.3**.

Table 3.11. Interventional therapy in stable COPD
Lung volume reduction surgery
• Lung volume reduction surgery improves survival in severe emphysema patients with an upper–lobe emphysema and low post–rehabilitation exercise capacity (**Evidence A**).
Bullectomy
• In selected patients bullectomy is associated with decreased dyspnea, improved lung function and exercise tolerance (**Evidence C**).
Transplantation
• In appropriately selected patients with very severe COPD, lung transplantation has been shown to improve quality of life and functional capacity (**Evidence C**).
Bronchoscopic interventions
• In select patients with advanced emphysema, bronchoscopic interventions reduces end-expiratory lung volume and improves exercise tolerance, health status and lung function at 6-12 months following treatment. Endobronchial valves (**Evidence B**); Lung coils (**Evidence B**).

Figure 4.3. Interventional Bronchoscopic and Surgical Treatments for COPD

Overview of various therapies used to treat patients with COPD and emphysema worldwide. Note that all therapies are not approved for clinical care in all countries. Additionally, the effects of BLVR on survival or other long term outcomes or comparison to LVRS are unknown.

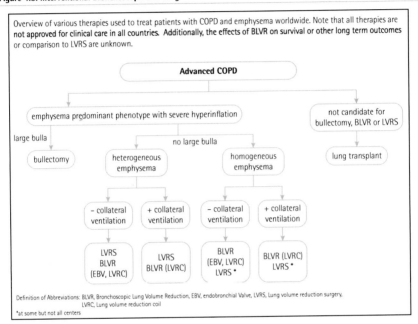

Definition of Abbreviations: BLVR, Bronchoscopic Lung Volume Reduction, EBV, endobronchial Valve, LVRS, Lung volume reduction surgery, LVRC, Lung volume reduction coil

*at some but not all centers

MANAGEMENT OF STABLE COPD

OVERALL KEY POINTS:

- *The management strategy for stable COPD should be predominantly based on the individualized assessment of symptoms and future risk of exacerbations.*

- *All individuals who smoke should be strongly encouraged and supported to quit.*

- *The main treatment goals are reduction of symptoms and future risk of exacerbations.*

- *Management strategies are not limited to pharmacological treatments, and should be complemented by appropriate non-pharmacological interventions.*

Once COPD has been diagnosed, effective management should be based on an individualized assessment to reduce both current symptoms and future risks of exacerbations (**Table 4.1**).

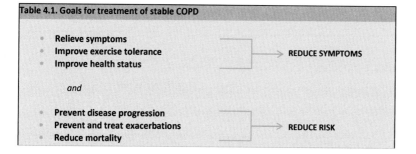

Table 4.1. Goals for treatment of stable COPD

- Relieve symptoms
- Improve exercise tolerance
- Improve health status

and

- Prevent disease progression
- Prevent and treat exacerbations
- Reduce mortality

REDUCE SYMPTOMS

REDUCE RISK

IDENTIFY AND REDUCE EXPOSURE TO RISK FACTORS

Identification and reduction of exposure to risk factors (**Table 4.2** and **4.3**) is important in the treatment and prevention of COPD. Cigarette smoking is the most commonly encountered and easily identifiable risk factor for COPD, and smoking cessation should be continually encouraged for all individuals who smoke. Reduction of total personal exposure to occupational dusts, fumes, and gases, and to indoor and outdoor air pollutants, should also be addressed.

Table 4.2. Treating tobacco use and dependence: A clinical practice guideline—major findings and recommendations

- Tobacco dependence is a chronic condition that warrants repeated treatment until long-term or permanent abstinence is achieved.
- Effective treatments for tobacco dependence exist and all tobacco users should be offered these treatments.
- Clinicians and health care delivery systems must operationalize the consistent identification, documentation, and treatment of every tobacco user at every visit.
- Brief smoking cessation counseling is effective and every tobacco user should be offered such advice at every contact with health care providers.
- There is a strong dose-response relation between the intensity of tobacco dependence counseling and its effectiveness.
- Three types of counseling have been found to be especially effective: practical counseling, social support of family and friends as part of treatment, and social support arranged outside of treatment.
- First-line pharmacotherapies for tobacco dependence—varenicline, bupropion sustained release, nicotine gum, nicotine inhaler, nicotine nasal spray, and nicotine patch—are effective and at least one of these medications should be prescribed in the absence of contraindications.
- Financial incentive programs for smoking cessation may facilitate smoking cessation.
- Tobacco dependence treatments are cost effective interventions.

Table 4.3. Identify and reduce risk factor exposure

- Smoking cessation interventions should be actively pursued in all COPD patients (**Evidence A**).
- Efficient ventilation, non-polluting cooking stoves and similar interventions should be recommended (**Evidence B**).
- Clinicians should advise patients to avoid continued exposures to potential irritants, if possible (**Evidence D**).

TREATMENT OF STABLE COPD

PHARMACOLOGIC TREATMENT

Pharmacologic therapies can reduce symptoms, and the risk and severity of exacerbations, as well as improve health status and exercise tolerance.

Most of the drugs are inhaled so proper inhaler technique is of high relevance. Key points for the inhalation of drugs are given in **Table 4.4**. Key points for bronchodilator use are given in **Table 4.5**. Key points for the use of anti-inflammatory agents are summarized in **Table 4.6**. Key points for the use of other pharmacologic treatments are summarized in **Table 4.7**.

Table 4.4. Key points for inhalation of drugs

- The choice of inhaler device has to be individually tailored and will depend on access, cost, prescriber, and most importantly, patient's ability and preference.
- It is essential to provide instructions and to demonstrate the proper inhalation technique when prescribing a device, to ensure that inhaler technique is adequate and re-check at each visit that patients continue to use their inhaler correctly.
- Inhaler technique (and adherence to therapy) should be assessed before concluding that the current therapy requires modification

Table 4.5. Key points for the use of bronchodilators

- LABAs and LAMAs are preferred over short-acting agents except for patients with only occasional dyspnea (**Evidence A**).
- Patients may be started on single long-acting bronchodilator therapy or dual long-acting bronchodilator therapy. In patients with persistent dyspnea on one bronchodilator treatment should be escalated to two (**Evidence A**).
- Inhaled bronchodilators are recommended over oral bronchodilators (**Evidence A**).
- Theophylline is not recommended unless other long-term treatment bronchodilators are unavailable or unaffordable (**Evidence B**).

Table 4.6. Key points for the use of anti-inflammatory agents

- Long-term monotherapy with ICS is not recommended (**Evidence A**).
- Long-term treatment with ICS may be considered in association with LABAs for patients with a history of exacerbations despite appropriate treatment with long-acting bronchodilators (**Evidence A**).
- Long-term therapy with oral corticosteroids is not recommended (**Evidence A**).
- In patients with exacerbations despite LABA/ICS or LABA/LAMA/ICS, chronic bronchitis and severe to very severe airflow obstruction, the addition of a PDE4 inhibitor can be considered (**Evidence B**).
- In former smokers with exacerbations despite appropriate therapy, macrolides can be considered (**Evidence B**).
- Statin therapy is not recommended for prevention of exacerbations (**Evidence A**).
- Antioxidant mucolytics are recommended only in selected patients (**Evidence A**).

Table 4.7. Key points for the use of other pharmacologic treatments

- Patients with severe hereditary alpha-1 antitrypsin deficiency and established emphysema may be candidates for alpha-1 antitrypsin augmentation therapy (**Evidence B**).
- Antitussives cannot be recommended (**Evidence C**).
- Drugs approved for primary pulmonary hypertension are not recommended for patients with pulmonary hypertension secondary to COPD (**Evidence B**).
- Low-dose long acting oral and parenteral opioids may be considered for treating dyspnea in COPD patients with severe disease (**Evidence B**).
- Review understanding of treatment regimen.

Pharmacologic treatment algorithms

A proposed model for the initiation, and then subsequent escalation and/or de-escalation of pharmacologic management of COPD according to the individualized assessment of symptoms and exacerbation risk is shown in **Figure 4.1**.

In past versions of the GOLD Report, recommendations were only given for initial therapy. However, many COPD patients are already on treatment and return with persistent symptoms after initial therapy, or less commonly with resolution of some symptoms that subsequently may require less therapy. Therefore, we now suggest escalation (and de-escalation) strategies. The recommendations made are based on available efficacy as well as safety data. We are fully aware that treatment escalation has not been systematically tested; trials of de-escalation are also limited and only include ICS.

These recommendations will be re-evaluated as additional data become available.

Figure 4.1. Pharmacologic treatment algorithms by GOLD Grade [highlighted boxes and arrows indicate preferred treatment pathways]

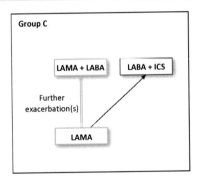

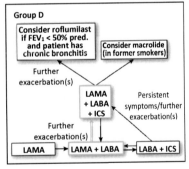

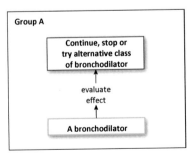

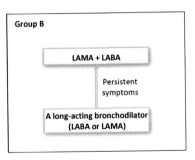

Preferred treatment = ⟹

In patients with a major discrepancy between the perceived level of symptoms and severity of airflow limitation, further evaluation is warranted.

Table 4.8. Non-pharmacologic management of COPD

Patient group	Essential	Recommended	Depending on local guidelines
A	Smoking cessation (can include pharmacologic treatment)	Physical activity	Flu vaccination Pneumococcal vaccination
B-D	Smoking cessation (can include pharmacologic treatment) Pulmonary rehabilitation	Physical activity	Flu vaccination Pneumococcal vaccination

Some relevant non-pharmacologic measures for patient groups A to D are summarized in **Table 4.8**. An appropriate algorithm for the prescription of oxygen to patients with COPD is shown in **Figure 4.2**.

Figure 4.2. Prescription of supplemental oxygen to COPD patients

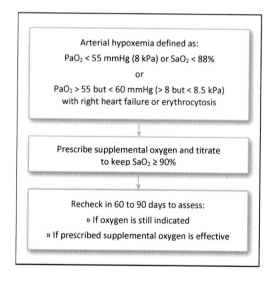

Arterial hypoxemia defined as:

$PaO_2 < 55$ mmHg (8 kPa) or $SaO_2 < 88\%$

or

$PaO_2 > 55$ but < 60 mmHg (> 8 but < 8.5 kPa) with right heart failure or erythrocytosis

Prescribe supplemental oxygen and titrate to keep $SaO_2 \geq 90\%$

Recheck in 60 to 90 days to assess:
» If oxygen is still indicated
» If prescribed supplemental oxygen is effective

Key points for the use of non-pharmacological treatments are given in **Table 4.9**.

Table 4.9. Key points for the use of non-pharmacological treatments

Education, self-management and pulmonary rehabilitation

- Education is needed to change patient's knowledge but there is no evidence that used alone it will change patient behavior.
- Education self-management with the support of a case manager with or without the use of a written action plan is recommended for the prevention of exacerbation complications such as hospital admissions (**Evidence B**).
- Rehabilitation is indicated in all patients with relevant symptoms and/or a high risk for exacerbation (**Evidence A**).
- Physical activity is a strong predictor of mortality (Evidence A). Patients should be encouraged to increase the level of physical activity although we still don't know how to best insure the likelihood of success.

Vaccination

- Influenza vaccination is recommended for all patients with COPD (**Evidence A**).
- Pneumococcal vaccination: the PCV13 and PPSV23 are recommended for all patients > 65 years of age, and in younger patients with significant comorbid conditions including chronic heart or lung disease (**Evidence B**).

Nutrition

- Nutritional supplementation should be considered in malnourished patients with COPD (**Evidence B**).

End of life and palliative care

- All clinicians managing patients with COPD should be aware of the effectiveness of palliative approaches to symptom control and use these in their practice (**Evidence D**).
- End of life care should include discussions with patients and their families about their views on resuscitation, advance directives and place of death preferences (**Evidence D**).

Treatment of hypoxemia

- In patients with severe resting hypoxemia long-term oxygen therapy is indicated (**Evidence A**).
- In patients with stable COPD and resting or exercise-induced moderate desaturation, long term oxygen treatment should not be routinely prescribed. However, individual patient factors may be considered when evaluating the patient's needs for supplemental oxygen (**Evidence A**).
- Resting oxygenation at sea level does not exclude the development of severe hypoxemia when travelling by air (**Evidence C**).

Treatment of hypercapnia

- In patients with severe chronic hypercapnia and a history of hospitalization for acute respiratory failure, long term non-invasive ventilation may be considered (**Evidence B**).

Intervention bronchoscopy and surgery

- Lung volume reduction surgery should be considered in selected patients with upper-lobe emphysema (**Evidence A**).
- Bronchoscopic lung volume reduction interventions may be considered in selected patients with advanced emphysema (**Evidence B**).
- In selected patients with a large bulla surgical bullectomy may be considered (**Evidence C**).
- In patients with very severe COPD (progressive disease, BODE score of 7 to 10, and not candidate for lung volume reduction) lung transplantation may be considered for referral with at least one of the following: (1) history of hospitalization for exacerbation associated with acute hypercapnia (Pco$_2$ > 50 mm Hg); (2) pulmonary hypertension and/or cor pulmonale, despite oxygen therapy; or (3) FEV$_1$ < 20% and either DLCO < 20% or homogenous distribution of emphysema (**Evidence C**).

MONITORING AND FOLLOW-UP

Routine follow-up of COPD patients is essential. Lung function may worsen over time, even with the best available care. Symptoms, exacerbations and objective measures of airflow limitation should be monitored to determine when to modify management and to identify any complications and/or comorbidities that may develop. Based on current literature, comprehensive self-management or routine monitoring has not shown long term benefits in terms of health status over usual care alone for COPD patients in general practice.[100]

MANAGEMENT OF EXACERBATIONS

OVERALL KEY POINTS:

- *An exacerbation of COPD is defined as an acute worsening of respiratory symptoms that results in additional therapy.*

- *Exacerbations of COPD can be precipitated by several factors. The most common causes are respiratory tract infections.*

- *The goal for treatment of COPD exacerbations is to minimize the negative impact of the current exacerbation and to prevent subsequent events.*

- *Short-acting inhaled beta$_2$-agonists, with or without short-acting anticholinergics, are recommended as the initial bronchodilators to treat an acute exacerbation.*

- *Maintenance therapy with long-acting bronchodilators should be initiated as soon as possible before hospital discharge.*

- *Systemic corticosteroids can improve lung function (FEV$_1$), oxygenation and shorten recovery time and hospitalization duration. Duration of therapy should not be more than 5-7 days.*

- *Antibiotics, when indicated, can shorten recovery time, reduce the risk of early relapse, treatment failure, and hospitalization duration. Duration of therapy should be 5-7 days.*

- *Methylxanthines are not recommended due to increased side effect profiles.*

- *Non-invasive mechanical ventilation should be the first mode of ventilation used in COPD patients with acute respiratory failure who have no absolute contraindication because it improves gas exchange, reduces work of breathing and the need for intubation, decreases hospitalization duration and improves survival.*

- *Following an exacerbation, appropriate measures for exacerbation prevention should be initiated (see Chapters 3 and 4 of GOLD 2017 full report).*

COPD exacerbations are defined as an acute worsening of respiratory symptoms that result in additional therapy.[101,102]

They are classified as:

- Mild (treated with short acting bronchodilators only, SABDs)
- Moderate (treated with SABDs plus antibiotics and/or oral corticosteroids) or
- Severe (patient requires hospitalization or visits the emergency room). Severe exacerbations may also be associated with acute respiratory failure.

Exacerbations of COPD are important events in the management of COPD because they negatively impact health status, rates of hospitalization and readmission, and disease progression.[101,102] COPD exacerbations are complex events usually associated with increased airway inflammation, increased mucous production and marked gas trapping. These changes contribute to increased dyspnea that is the key symptom of an exacerbation. Other symptoms include increased sputum purulence and volume, together with increased cough and wheeze.[103] As co-morbidities are common in COPD patients, exacerbations must be differentiated clinically from other events such as acute coronary syndrome, worsening congestive heart failure, pulmonary embolism and pneumonia.

TREATMENT OPTIONS

Treatment Setting

The goals of treatment for COPD exacerbations are to minimize the negative impact of the current exacerbation and prevent the development of subsequent events.[104] Depending on the severity of an exacerbation and/or the severity of the underlying disease, an exacerbation can be managed in either the outpatient or inpatient setting. More than 80% of exacerbations are managed on an outpatient basis with pharmacologic therapies including bronchodilators, corticosteroids, and antibiotics.[15,23,24]

The clinical presentation of COPD exacerbation is heterogeneous, thus we recommend that in **hospitalized patients** the severity of the exacerbation should be based on the patient's clinical signs and recommend the following classification.[105]

No respiratory failure: Respiratory rate: 20-30 breaths per minute; no use of accessory respiratory muscles; no changes in mental status; hypoxemia improved with supplemental oxygen given via Venturi mask 28-35% inspired oxygen (FiO_2); no increase in $PaCO_2$.

Acute respiratory failure — non-life-threatening: Respiratory rate: > 30 breaths per minute; using accessory respiratory muscles; no change in mental status; hypoxemia improved with supplemental oxygen via Venturi mask 25-30% FiO_2; hypercarbia i.e., $PaCO_2$ increased compared with baseline or elevated 50-60 mmHg.

Acute respiratory failure — life-threatening: Respiratory rate: > 30 breaths per minute; using accessory respiratory muscles; acute changes in mental status; hypoxemia not improved with supplemental oxygen via Venturi mask or requiring FiO_2 > 40%; hypercarbia i.e., $PaCO_2$ increased compared with baseline or elevated > 60 mmHg or the presence of acidosis (pH $\leq$ 7.25).

Table 5.1. Potential indications for hospitalization assessment*

- Severe symptoms such as sudden worsening of resting dyspnea, high respiratory rate, decreased oxygen saturation, confusion, drowsiness.
- Acute respiratory failure.
- Onset of new physical signs (e.g., cyanosis, peripheral edema).
- Failure of an exacerbation to respond to initial medical management.
- Presence of serious comorbidities (e.g., heart failure, newly occurring arrhythmias, etc.).
- Insufficient home support.

*Local resources need to be considered.

Table 5.2. Management of severe but not life-threatening exacerbations*

- Assess severity of symptoms, blood gases, chest radiograph.
- Administer supplemental oxygen therapy, obtain serial arterial blood gas, venous blood gas and pulse oximetry measurements.
- Bronchodilators:
  - » Increase doses and/or frequency of short-acting bronchodilators.
  - » Combine short-acting beta 2-agonists and anticholinergics.
  - » Consider use of long-active bronchodilators when patient becomes stable.
  - » Use spacers or air-driven nebulizers when appropriate.
- Consider oral corticosteroids.
- Consider antibiotics (oral) when signs of bacterial infection are present.
- Consider noninvasive mechanical ventilation (NIV).
- At all times:
  - » Monitor fluid balance.
  - » Consider subcutaneous heparin or low molecular weight heparin for thromboembolism prophylaxis.
  - » Identify and treat associated conditions (e.g., heart failure, arrhythmias, pulmonary embolism etc.).

*Local resources need to be considered.

The indications for assessing the need for hospitalization during a COPD exacerbation are shown in **Table 5.1**. When patients with a COPD exacerbation come to the emergency department, they should be provided with supplemental oxygen and undergo assessment to determine whether the exacerbation is life-threatening and if increased work of breathing or impaired gas exchange requires consideration for non-invasive ventilation. The management of severe, but not life threatening, exacerbations is outlined in **Table 5.2**.

Key points for the management of exacerbations are given in **Table 5.3**.

Table 5.3. Key points for the management of exacerbations

• Short-acting inhaled beta$_2$-agonists, with or without short-acting anticholinergics, are recommended as the initial bronchodilators to treat an acute exacerbation **(Evidence C)**.

• Systemic corticosteroids can improve lung function (FEV$_1$), oxygenation and shorten recovery time and hospitalization duration. Duration of therapy should not be more than 5-7 days **(Evidence A)**.

• Antibiotics, when indicated, can shorten recovery time, reduce the risk of early relapse, treatment failure, and hospitalization duration. Duration of therapy should be 5-7 days **(Evidence B)**.

• Methylxanthines are not recommended due to increased side effect profiles **(Evidence B)**.

• Non-invasive mechanical ventilation should be the first mode of ventilation used in COPD patients with acute respiratory failure **(Evidence A)**.

• NIV should be the first mode of ventilation used in COPD patients with acute respiratory failure who have no absolute contraindication because it improves gas exchange, reduces work of breathing and the need for intubation, decreases hospitalization duration and improves survival **(Evidence A)**.

Table 5.4. Indications for respiratory or medical intensive care unit admission*

• Severe dyspnea that responds inadequately to initial emergency therapy.

• Changes in mental status (confusion, lethargy, coma).

• Persistent or worsening hypoxemia (PaO$_2$ < 5.3 kPa or 40 mmHg) and/or severe/worsening respiratory acidosis (pH < 7.25) despite supplemental oxygen and noninvasive ventilation.

• Need for invasive mechanical ventilation.

• Hemodynamic instability—need for vasopressors.

*Local resources need to be considered.

Noninvasive mechanical ventilation

• The use of noninvasive mechanical ventilation (NIV) is preferred over invasive ventilation (intubation and positive pressure ventilation) as the initial mode of ventilation to treat acute respiratory failure in patients hospitalized for acute exacerbations of COPD.

• The indications for NIV[108] are summarized in **Table 5.5**.

Table 5.5. Indications for noninvasive mechanical ventilation (NIV)

At least one of the following:

• Respiratory acidosis (PaCO$_2$ ≥ 6.0 kPa or 45 mmHg and arterial pH ≤ 7.35).

• Severe dyspnea with clinical signs suggestive of respiratory muscle fatigue, increased work of breathing, or both, such as use of respiratory accessory muscles, paradoxical motion of the abdomen, or retraction of the intercostal spaces.

• Persistent hypoxemia despite supplemental oxygen therapy.

Table 5.6. Indications for invasive mechanical ventilation
• Unable to tolerate NIV or NIV failure.
• Status post - respiratory or cardiac arrest.
• Diminished consciousness, psychomotor agitation inadequately controlled by sedation.
• Massive aspiration or persistent vomiting.
• Persistent inability to remove respiratory secretions.
• Severe hemodynamic instability without response to fluids and vasoactive drugs.
• Severe ventricular or supraventricular arrhythmias.
• Life-threatening hypoxemia in patients unable to tolerate NIV.

Invasive mechanical ventilation. The indications for initiating invasive mechanical ventilation during an exacerbation are shown in **Table 5.6,** and include failure of an initial trial of NIV.[109]
Prevention of exacerbations

HOSPITAL DISCHARGE AND FOLLOW-UP

Early follow-up (within one month) following discharge should be undertaken when possible and has been related to less exacerbation-related readmissions.[110] A review of discharge criter and recommendations for follow-up are summarized in **Table 5.7**.

Table 5.7. Discharge criteria and recommendations for follow-up
● Full review of all clinical and laboratory data.
● Check maintenance therapy and understanding.
● Reassess inhaler technique.
● Ensure understanding of withdrawal of acute medications (steroids and/or antibiotics).
● Assess need for continuing any oxygen therapy.
● Provide management plan for comorbidities and follow-up.
● Ensure follow-up arrangements: early follow-up < 4 weeks, and late follow-up < 12 weeks as indicated.
● All clinical or investigational abnormalities have been identified.
1–4 Weeks Follow-Up
● Evaluate ability to cope in his/her usual environment.
● Review and understanding treatment regimen.
● Reassessment of inhaler techniques.
● Reassess need for long-term oxygen.
● Document the capacity to do physical activity and activities of daily living.
● Document symptoms: CAT or mMRC.
● Determine status of comorbidities.
12–16 Weeks Follow-Up
● Evaluate ability to cope in his/her usual environment.
● Review understanding treatment regimen.
● Reassessment of inhaler techniques.
● Reassess need for long-term oxygen.
● Document the capacity to do physical activity and activities of daily living.
● Measure spirometry: FEV_1.
● Document symptoms: CAT or mMRC.
● Determine status of comorbidities.

After an acute exacerbation appropriate measures for prevention of further exacerbations should be initiated (**Table 5.8**).

Table 5.8. Interventions that reduce the frequency of COPD exacerbations	
Intervention class	**Intervention**
Bronchodilators	LABAs LAMAs LABA + LAMA
Corticosteroid-containing regimens	LABA + ICS LABA + LAMA + ICS
Anti-inflammatory (non-steroid)	Roflumilast
Anti-infectives	Vaccines Long term macrolides
Mucoregulators	N-acetylcysteine Carbocysteine
Various others	Smoking cessation Rehabilitation Lung volume reduction

COPD AND COMORBIDITIES

OVERALL KEY POINTS:

- COPD often coexists with other diseases (comorbidities) that may have a significant impact on disease course.

- In general, the presence of comorbidities should not alter COPD treatment and comorbidities should be treated per usual standards regardless of the presence of COPD.

- Lung cancer is frequently seen in patients with COPD and is a main cause of death.

- Cardiovascular diseases are common and important comorbidities in COPD

- Osteoporosis, depression/anxiety, and obstructive sleep apnea are frequent, important comorbidities in COPD, are often under-diagnosed, and are associated with poor health status and prognosis.

- Gastroesophageal reflux (GERD) is associated with an increased risk of exacerbations and poorer health status.

- When COPD is part of a multimorbidity care plan, attention should be directed to ensure simplicity of treatment and to minimize polypharmacy.

REFERENCES

1. Lozano R, Naghavi M, Foreman K, et al. Global and regional mortality from 235 causes of death for 20 age groups in 1990 and 2010: a systematic analysis for the Global Burden of Disease Study 2010. *Lancet* 2012; **380**(9859): 2095-128.

2. Mathers CD, Loncar D. Projections of global mortality and burden of disease from 2002 to 2030. *PLoS Med* 2006; **3**(11): e442.

3. Lange P, Celli B, Agusti A, et al. Lung-Function Trajectories Leading to Chronic Obstructive Pulmonary Disease. *N Engl J Med* 2015; **373**(2): 111-22.

4. Stern DA, Morgan WJ, Wright AL, Guerra S, Martinez FD. Poor airway function in early infancy and lung function by age 22 years: a non-selective longitudinal cohort study. *Lancet* 2007; **370**(9589): 758-64.

5. Tashkin DP, Altose MD, Bleecker ER, et al. The lung health study: airway responsiveness to inhaled methacholine in smokers with mild to moderate airflow limitation. The Lung Health Study Research Group. *Am Rev Respir Dis* 1992; **145**(2 Pt 1): 301-10.

6. Eisner MD, Anthonisen N, Coultas D, et al. An official American Thoracic Society public policy statement: Novel risk factors and the global burden of chronic obstructive pulmonary disease. *Am J Respir Crit Care Med* 2010; **182**(5): 693-718.

7. Salvi SS, Barnes PJ. Chronic obstructive pulmonary disease in non-smokers. *Lancet* 2009; **374**(9691): 733-43.

8. Paulin LM, Diette GB, Blanc PD, et al. Occupational exposures are associated with worse morbidity in patients with chronic obstructive pulmonary disease. *Am J Respir Crit Care Med* 2015; **191**(5): 557-65.

9. Stoller JK, Aboussouan LS. Alpha1-antitrypsin deficiency. *Lancet* 2005; **365**(9478): 2225-36.

10. Gershon AS, Warner L, Cascagnette P, Victor JC, To T. Lifetime risk of developing chronic obstructive pulmonary disease: a longitudinal population study. *Lancet* 2011; **378**(9795): 991-6.

11. de Marco R, Accordini S, Marcon A, et al. Risk factors for chronic obstructive pulmonary disease in a European cohort of young adults. *Am J Respir Crit Care Med* 2011; **183**(7): 891-7

12. Buist AS, McBurnie MA, Vollmer WM, et al. International variation in the prevalence of COPD (the BOLD Study): a population-based prevalence study. *Lancet* 2007; **370**(9589): 741-50.

13. Jackson H, Hubbard R. Detecting chronic obstructive pulmonary disease using peak flow rate: cross sectional survey. *BMJ* 2003; **327**(7416): 653-4.

14. WHO meeting participants. Alpha 1-antitrypsin deficiency: memorandum from a WHO meeting. *Bull World Health Organ* 1997; **75**(5): 397-415.

15. Jones PW. Health status and the spiral of decline. *COPD* 2009; **6**(1): 59-63.

16. Han MK, Muellerova H, Curran-Everett D, et al. GOLD 2011 disease severity classification in COPDGene: a prospective cohort study. *The Lancet Respiratory medicine* 2013; **1**(1): 43-50.

17. Fletcher CM. Standardised questionnaire on respiratory symptoms: a statement prepared and approved by the MRC Committee on the Aetiology of Chronic Bronchitis (MRC breathlessness score). *BMJ* 1960; **2**: 1662.

18. Sundh J, Janson C, Lisspers K, Stallberg B, Montgomery S. The Dyspnoea, Obstruction, Smoking, Exacerbation (DOSE) index is predictive of mortality in COPD. *Prim Care Respir J* 2012; **21**(3): 295-301.

19. Nishimura K, Izumi T, Tsukino M, Oga T. Dyspnea is a better predictor of 5-year survival than airway obstruction in patients with COPD. *Chest* 2002; **121**(5): 1434-40.

20. Jones PW. Health status measurement in chronic obstructive pulmonary disease. *Thorax* 2001; **56**(11): 880-7.

21. Soriano JB, Lamprecht B, Ramirez AS, et al. Mortality prediction in chronic obstructive pulmonary disease comparing the GOLD 2007 and 2011 staging systems: a pooled analysis of individual patient data. *The Lancet Respiratory medicine* 2015; **3**(6): 443-50.

22. Goossens LM, Leimer I, Metzdorf N, Becker K, Rutten-van Molken MP. Does the 2013 GOLD classification improve the ability to predict lung function decline, exacerbations and mortality: a post-hoc analysis of the 4-year UPLIFT trial. *BMC Pulm Med* 2014; **14**: 163.

23. Kim J, Yoon HI, Oh YM, et al. Lung function decline rates according to GOLD group in patients with chronic obstructive pulmonary disease. *Int J Chron Obstruct Pulmon Dis* 2015; **10**: 1819-27.

24. van Eerd EA, van der Meer RM, van Schayck OC, Kotz D. Smoking cessation for people with chronic obstructive pulmonary disease. *Cochrane Database Syst Rev* 2016; (8): CD010744.

25. The Tobacco Use and Dependence Clinical Practice Guideline Panel. A clinical practice guideline for treating tobacco use and dependence: A US Public Health Service report. *JAMA* 2000; **283**(24): 3244-54.

26. The tobacco use and dependence clinical practice guideline panel s, and consortium representatives,. A clinical practice guideline for treating tobacco use and dependence. *JAMA* 2000; **28**: 3244-54.

27. U.S. Public Health Service. A clinical practice guideline for treating tobacco use and dependence: 2008 update. A U.S. Public Health Service report. *American journal of preventive medicine* 2008; **35**(2): 158-76.

28. Glynn T, Manley M. How to help your patients stop smoking. A National Cancer Institute manual for physicians. In: U.S. Department of Health and Human Services PHS, National Institutes of Health, National Cancer Institute., editor.; 1990.

29. Stead LF, Buitrago D, Preciado N, Sanchez G, Hartmann-Boyce J, Lancaster T. Physician advice for smoking cessation. *Cochrane Database Syst Rev* 2013; **5**(5): CD000165.

30. Kottke TE, Battista RN, DeFriese GH, Brekke ML. Attributes of successful smoking cessation interventions in medical practice. A meta-analysis of 39 controlled trials. *JAMA* 1988; **259**(19): 2883-9.

31. Wongsurakiat P, Maranetra KN, Wasi C, Kositanont U, Dejsomritrutai W, Charoenratanakul S. Acute respiratory illness in patients with COPD and the effectiveness of influenza vaccination: a randomized controlled study. *Chest* 2004; **125**(6): 2011-20.

32. Poole PJ, Chacko E, Wood-Baker RW, Cates CJ. Influenza vaccine for patients with chronic obstructive pulmonary disease. *Cochrane Database Syst Rev* 2006; (1): CD002733.

33. Wongsurakiat P, Lertakyamanee J, Maranetra KN, Jongriratanakul S, Sangkaew S. Economic evaluation of influenza vaccination in Thai chronic obstructive pulmonary disease patients. *J Med Assoc Thai* 2003; **86**(6): 497-508.

34. Nichol KL, Margolis KL, Wuorenma J, Von Sternberg T. The efficacy and cost effectiveness of vaccination against influenza among elderly persons living in the community. *N Engl J Med* 1994; **331**(12): 778-84.

35. Fiore AE, Shay DK, Broder K, et al. Prevention and control of seasonal influenza with vaccines: recommendations of the Advisory Committee on Immunization Practices (ACIP), 2009. *MMWR Recomm Rep* 2009; **58**(RR-8): 1-52.

36. Tomczyk S, Bennett NM, Stoecker C, et al. Use of 13-valent pneumococcal conjugate vaccine and 23-valent pneumococcal polysaccharide vaccine among adults aged >/=65 years: recommendations of the Advisory Committee on Immunization Practices (ACIP). *MMWR Morb Mortal Wkly Rep* 2014; **63**(37): 822-5.

37. Alfageme I, Vazquez R, Reyes N, et al. Clinical efficacy of anti-pneumococcal vaccination in patients with COPD. *Thorax* 2006; **61**(3): 189-95.

38. Burge PS, Calverley PM, Jones PW, Spencer S, Anderson JA, Maslen TK. Randomised, double blind, placebo controlled study of fluticasone propionate in patients with moderate to severe chronic obstructive pulmonary disease: the ISOLDE trial. *BMJ* 2000; **320**(7245): 1297-303.

39. Anthonisen NR, Connett JE, Kiley JP, et al. Effects of smoking intervention and the use of an inhaled anticholinergic bronchodilator on the rate of decline of FEV1. The Lung Health Study. *JAMA* 1994; **272**(19): 1497-505.

40. Pauwels RA, Lofdahl CG, Laitinen LA, et al. Long-term treatment with inhaled budesonide in persons with mild chronic obstructive pulmonary disease who continue smoking. European Respiratory Society Study on Chronic Obstructive Pulmonary Disease. *N Engl J Med* 1999; **340**(25): 1948-53.

41. Vestbo J, Sorensen T, Lange P, Brix A, Torre P, Viskum K. Long-term effect of inhaled budesonide in mild and moderate chronic obstructive pulmonary disease: a randomised controlled trial. *Lancet* 1999; **353**(9167): 1819-23.

42. Tashkin DP, Celli B, Senn S, et al. A 4-year trial of tiotropium in chronic obstructive pulmonary disease. *N Engl J Med* 2008; **359**(15): 1543-54.

43. Kew KM, Mavergames C, Walters JA. Long-acting beta2-agonists for chronic obstructive pulmonary disease. *Cochrane Database Syst Rev* 2013; **10**(10): CD010177.

44. Han J, Dai L, Zhong N. Indacaterol on dyspnea in chronic obstructive pulmonary disease: a systematic review and meta-analysis of randomized placebo-controlled trials. *BMC Pulm Med* 2013; **13**: 26.

45. Geake JB, Dabscheck EJ, Wood-Baker R, Cates CJ. Indacaterol, a once-daily beta2-agonist, versus twice-daily beta(2)-agonists or placebo for chronic obstructive pulmonary disease. *Cochrane Database Syst Rev* 2015; **1**: CD010139.

46. Koch A, Pizzichini E, Hamilton A, et al. Lung function efficacy and symptomatic benefit of olodaterol once daily delivered via Respimat(R) versus placebo and formoterol twice daily in patients with GOLD 2-4 COPD: results from two replicate 48-week studies. *Int J Chron Obstruct Pulmon Dis* 2014; **9**: 697-714.

47. Kempsford R, Norris V, Siederer S. Vilanterol trifenatate, a novel inhaled long-acting beta2 adrenoceptor agonist, is well tolerated in healthy subjects and demonstrates prolonged bronchodilation in subjects with asthma and COPD. *Pulm Pharmacol Ther* 2013; **26**(2): 256-64.

48. Melani AS. Long-acting muscarinic antagonists. *Expert Rev Clin Pharmacol* 2015; **8**(4): 479-501.

49. Appleton S, Jones T, Poole P, et al. Ipratropium bromide versus long-acting beta-2 agonists for stable chronic obstructive pulmonary disease. *Cochrane Database Syst Rev* 2006; (3): Cd006101.

50. Vogelmeier C, Hederer B, Glaab T, et al. Tiotropium versus salmeterol for the prevention of exacerbations of COPD. *N Engl J Med* 2011; **364**(12): 1093-103.

51. Decramer ML, Chapman KR, Dahl R, et al. Once-daily indacaterol versus tiotropium for patients with severe chronic obstructive pulmonary disease (INVIGORATE): a randomised, blinded, parallel-group study. *The Lancet Respiratory medicine* 2013; **1**(7): 524-33.

52. Tashkin DP. Long-acting anticholinergic use in chronic obstructive pulmonary disease: efficacy and safety. *Curr Opin Pulm Med* 2010; **16**(2): 97-105.

53. Disse B, Speck GA, Rominger KL, Witek TJ, Jr., Hammer R. Tiotropium (Spiriva): mechanistical considerations and clinical profile in obstructive lung disease. *Life Sci* 1999; **64**(6-7): 457-64.

54. Barnes P. Bronchodilators: basic pharmacology. In: Calverley PMA, Pride NB, eds. Chronic obstructive pulmonary disease. London: Chapman and Hall; 1995: 391-417.

55. Ram FS, Jones PW, Castro AA, et al. Oral theophylline for chronic obstructive pulmonary disease. *Cochrane Database Syst Rev* 2002; (4): CD003902.

56. ZuWallack RL, Mahler DA, Reilly D, et al. Salmeterol plus theophylline combination therapy in the treatment of COPD. *Chest* 2001; **119**(6): 1661-70.

57. Zacarias EC, Castro AA, Cendon S. Effect of theophylline associated with short-acting or long-acting inhaled beta2-agonists in patients with stable chronic obstructive pulmonary disease: a systematic review. *J Bras Pneumol* 2007; **33**(2): 152-60.

58. Cosio BG, Shafiek H, Iglesias A, et al. Oral Low-dose Theophylline on Top of Inhaled Fluticasone-Salmeterol Does Not Reduce Exacerbations in Patients With Severe COPD: A Pilot Clinical Trial. *Chest* 2016; **150**(1): 123-30.

59. Zhou Y, Wang X, Zeng X, et al. Positive benefits of theophylline in a randomized, double-blind, parallel-group, placebo-controlled study of low-dose, slow-release theophylline in the treatment of COPD for 1 year. *Respirology* 2006; **11**(5): 603-10.

60. McKay SE, Howie CA, Thomson AH, Whiting B, Addis GJ. Value of theophylline treatment in patients handicapped by chronic obstructive lung disease. *Thorax* 1993; **48**(3): 227-32.

61. Cazzola M, Molimard M. The scientific rationale for combining long-acting beta2-agonists and muscarinic antagonists in COPD. *Pulm Pharmacol Ther* 2010; **23**(4): 257-67.

62. Gross N, Tashkin D, Miller R, Oren J, Coleman W, Linberg S. Inhalation by nebulization of albuterol-ipratropium combination (Dey combination) is superior to either agent alone in the treatment of chronic obstructive pulmonary disease. Dey Combination Solution Study Group. *Respiration* 1998; **65**(5): 354-62.

63. Tashkin DP, Pearle J, Iezzoni D, Varghese ST. Formoterol and tiotropium compared with tiotropium alone for treatment of COPD. *COPD* 2009; **6**(1): 17-25.

64. Mahler DA, Kerwin E, Ayers T, et al. FLIGHT1 and FLIGHT2: Efficacy and Safety of QVA149 (Indacaterol/Glycopyrrolate) versus Its Monocomponents and Placebo in Patients with Chronic Obstructive Pulmonary Disease. *Am J Respir Crit Care Med* 2015; **192**(9): 1068-79.

65. Nannini LJ, Lasserson TJ, Poole P. Combined corticosteroid and long-acting beta(2)-agonist in one inhaler versus long-acting beta(2)-agonists for chronic obstructive pulmonary disease. *Cochrane Database Syst Rev* 2012; **9**(9): CD006829.

66. Nannini LJ, Poole P, Milan SJ, Kesterton A. Combined corticosteroid and long-acting beta(2)-agonist in one inhaler versus inhaled corticosteroids alone for chronic obstructive pulmonary disease. *Cochrane Database Syst Rev* 2013; **8**(8): CD006826.

67. Yang IA, Clarke MS, Sim EH, Fong KM. Inhaled corticosteroids for stable chronic obstructive pulmonary disease. *Cochrane Database Syst Rev* 2012; **7**(7): CD002991.

68. Nadeem NJ, Taylor SJ, Eldridge SM. Withdrawal of inhaled corticosteroids in individuals with COPD--a systematic review and comment on trial methodology. *Respir Res* 2011; **12**: 107.

69. van der Valk P, Monninkhof E, van der Palen J, Zielhuis G, van Herwaarden C. Effect of discontinuation of inhaled corticosteroids in patients with chronic obstructive pulmonary disease: the COPE study. *Am J Respir Crit Care Med* 2002; **166**(10): 1358-63.

70. Wouters EF, Postma DS, Fokkens B, et al. Withdrawal of fluticasone propionate from combined salmeterol/fluticasone treatment in patients with COPD causes immediate and sustained disease deterioration: a randomised controlled trial. *Thorax* 2005; **60**(6): 480-7.

71. Kunz LI, Postma DS, Klooster K, et al. Relapse in FEV1 Decline After Steroid Withdrawal in COPD. *Chest* 2015; **148**(2): 389-96.

72. Magnussen H, Disse B, Rodriguez-Roisin R, et al. Withdrawal of inhaled glucocorticoids and exacerbations of COPD. *N Engl J Med* 2014; **371**(14): 1285-94.

73. Brusselle G, Price D, Gruffydd-Jones K, et al. The inevitable drift to triple therapy in COPD: an analysis of prescribing pathways in the UK. *Int J Chron Obstruct Pulmon Dis* 2015; **10**: 2207-17.

74. Welte T, Miravitlles M, Hernandez P, et al. Efficacy and tolerability of budesonide/formoterol added to tiotropium in patients with chronic obstructive pulmonary disease. *Am J Respir Crit Care Med* 2009; **180**(8): 741-50.

75. Singh D, Brooks J, Hagan G, Cahn A, O'Connor BJ. Superiority of "triple" therapy with salmeterol/fluticasone propionate and tiotropium bromide versus individual components in moderate to severe COPD. *Thorax* 2008; **63**(7): 592-8.

76. Jung KS, Park HY, Park SY, et al. Comparison of tiotropium plus fluticasone propionate/salmeterol with tiotropium in COPD: a randomized controlled study. *Respir Med* 2012; **106**(3): 382-9.

77. Hanania NA, Crater GD, Morris AN, Emmett AH, O'Dell DM, Niewoehner DE. Benefits of adding fluticasone propionate/salmeterol to tiotropium in moderate to severe COPD. *Respir Med* 2012; **106**(1): 91-101.

78. Frith PA, Thompson PJ, Ratnavadivel R, et al. Glycopyrronium once-daily significantly improves lung function and health status when combined with salmeterol/fluticasone in patients with COPD: the GLISTEN study, a randomised controlled trial. *Thorax* 2015; **70**(6): 519-27.

79. Siler TM, Kerwin E, Singletary K, Brooks J, Church A. Efficacy and Safety of Umeclidinium Added to Fluticasone Propionate/Salmeterol in Patients with COPD: Results of Two Randomized, Double-Blind Studies. *COPD* 2016; **13**(1): 1-10.

80. Singh D, Papi A, Corradi M, et al. Single inhaler triple therapy versus inhaled corticosteroid plus long-acting beta2-agonist therapy for chronic obstructive pulmonary disease (TRILOGY): a double-blind, parallel group, randomised controlled trial. *Lancet* 2016; **388**(10048): 963-73.

81. Aaron SD, Vandemheen KL, Fergusson D, et al. Tiotropium in combination with placebo, salmeterol, or fluticasone-salmeterol for treatment of chronic obstructive pulmonary disease: a randomized trial. *Ann Intern Med* 2007; **146**(8): 545-55.

82. Manson SC, Brown RE, Cerulli A, Vidaurre CF. The cumulative burden of oral corticosteroid side effects and the economic implications of steroid use. *Respir Med* 2009; **103**(7): 975-94.

83. Calverley PM, Rabe KF, Goehring UM, et al. Roflumilast in symptomatic chronic obstructive pulmonary disease: two randomised clinical trials. *Lancet* 2009; **374**(9691): 685-94.

84. Chong J, Leung B, Poole P. Phosphodiesterase 4 inhibitors for chronic obstructive pulmonary disease. *Cochrane Database Syst Rev* 2013; **11**(11): CD002309.

85. Herath SC, Poole P. Prophylactic antibiotic therapy for chronic obstructive pulmonary disease (COPD). *Cochrane Database Syst Rev* 2013; (11): CD009764.

86. Ni W, Shao X, Cai X, et al. Prophylactic use of macrolide antibiotics for the prevention of chronic obstructive pulmonary disease exacerbation: a meta-analysis. *PloS one* 2015; **10**(3): e0121257.

87. Cazzola M, Calzetta L, Page C, et al. Influence of N-acetylcysteine on chronic bronchitis or COPD exacerbations: a meta-analysis. *Eur Respir Rev* 2015; **24**(137): 451-61.

88. Poole P, Chong J, Cates CJ. Mucolytic agents versus placebo for chronic bronchitis or chronic obstructive pulmonary disease. *Cochrane Database Syst Rev* 2015; (7): CD001287.

89. Rootmensen GN, van Keimpema AR, Jansen HM, de Haan RJ. Predictors of incorrect inhalation technique in patients with asthma or COPD: a study using a validated videotaped scoring method. *J Aerosol Med Pulm Drug Deliv* 2010; **23**(5): 323-8.

90. Sulaiman I, Cushen B, Greene G, et al. Objective Assessment of Adherence to Inhalers by COPD Patients. *Am J Respir Crit Care Med* 2016; **EPub 13 July 2016**.

91. McCarthy B, Casey D, Devane D, Murphy K, Murphy E, Lacasse Y. Pulmonary rehabilitation for chronic obstructive pulmonary disease. *Cochrane Database Syst Rev* 2015; **2**(2): CD003793.

92. Cranston JM, Crockett AJ, Moss JR, Alpers JH. Domiciliary oxygen for chronic obstructive pulmonary disease. *Cochrane Database Syst Rev* 2005; (4): CD001744.

93. Elliott MW, Nava S. Noninvasive ventilation for acute exacerbations of chronic obstructive pulmonary disease: "Don't think twice, it's alright!". *Am J Respir Crit Care Med* 2012; **185**(2): 121-3.

94.   Chandra D, Stamm JA, Taylor B, et al. Outcomes of noninvasive ventilation for acute exacerbations of chronic obstructive pulmonary disease in the United States, 1998-2008. *Am J Respir Crit Care Med* 2012; **185**(2): 152-9.

95.   Lindenauer PK, Stefan MS, Shieh MS, Pekow PS, Rothberg MB, Hill NS. Outcomes associated with invasive and noninvasive ventilation among patients hospitalized with exacerbations of chronic obstructive pulmonary disease. *JAMA Intern Med* 2014; **174**(12): 1982-93.

96.   Kohnlein T, Windisch W, Kohler D, et al. Non-invasive positive pressure ventilation for the treatment of severe stable chronic obstructive pulmonary disease: a prospective, multicentre, randomised, controlled clinical trial. *The Lancet Respiratory medicine* 2014; **2**(9): 698-705.

97.   Galli JA, Krahnke JS, James Mamary A, Shenoy K, Zhao H, Criner GJ. Home non-invasive ventilation use following acute hypercapnic respiratory failure in COPD. *Respir Med* 2014; **108**(5): 722-8.

98.   Coughlin S, Liang WE, Parthasarathy S. Retrospective Assessment of Home Ventilation to Reduce Rehospitalization in Chronic Obstructive Pulmonary Disease. *Journal of clinical sleep medicine : JCSM : official publication of the American Academy of Sleep Medicine* 2015; **11**(6): 663-70.

99.   Marin JM, Soriano JB, Carrizo SJ, Boldova A, Celli BR. Outcomes in patients with chronic obstructive pulmonary disease and obstructive sleep apnea: the overlap syndrome. *Am J Respir Crit Care Med* 2010; **182**(3): 325-31.

100.   Bischoff EW, Akkermans R, Bourbeau J, van Weel C, Vercoulen JH, Schermer TR. Comprehensive self management and routine monitoring in chronic obstructive pulmonary disease patients in general practice: randomised controlled trial. *BMJ* 2012; **345**: e7642.

101.   Wedzicha JA, Seemungal TA. COPD exacerbations: defining their cause and prevention. *Lancet* 2007; **370**(9589): 786-96.

102.   Seemungal TA, Donaldson GC, Paul EA, Bestall JC, Jeffries DJ, Wedzicha JA. Effect of exacerbation on quality of life in patients with chronic obstructive pulmonary disease. *Am J Respir Crit Care Med* 1998; **157**(5 Pt 1): 1418-22.

103.   Anthonisen NR, Manfreda J, Warren CP, Hershfield ES, Harding GK, Nelson NA. Antibiotic therapy in exacerbations of chronic obstructive pulmonary disease. *Ann Intern Med* 1987; **106**(2): 196-204.

104.   Martinez FI, Han MK, Flaherty K, Curtis J. Role of infection and antimicrobial therapy in acute exacerbations of chronic obstructive pulmonary disease. *Expert Rev Anti Infect Ther* 2006; **4**(1): 101-24.

105.   Celli BR, Barnes PJ. Exacerbations of chronic obstructive pulmonary disease. *Eur Respir J* 2007; **29**(6): 1224-38.

106.   Austin MA, Wills KE, Blizzard L, Walters EH, Wood-Baker R. Effect of high flow oxygen on mortality in chronic obstructive pulmonary disease patients in prehospital setting: randomised controlled trial. *BMJ* 2010; **341**: c5462.

107.   National Institute for Health and Care Excellence. Chronic obstructive pulmonary disease in over 16s: diagnosis and management. 2010. https://www.nice.org.uk/guidance/CG101.

108.   Consensus development conference committee. Clinical indications for noninvasive positive pressure ventilation in chronic respiratory failure due to restrictive lung disease, COPD, and nocturnal hypoventilation--a consensus conference report. *Chest* 1999; **116**(2): 521-34.

109.   Conti G, Antonelli M, Navalesi P, et al. Noninvasive vs. conventional mechanical ventilation in patients with chronic obstructive pulmonary disease after failure of medical treatment in the ward: a randomized trial. *Intensive Care Med* 2002; **28**(12): 1701-7.

110.   Gavish R, Levy A, Dekel OK, Karp E, Maimon N. The Association Between Hospital Readmission and Pulmonologist Follow-up Visits in Patients With COPD. *Chest* 2015; **148**(2): 375-81.

Made in the USA
Lexington, KY
12 April 2018